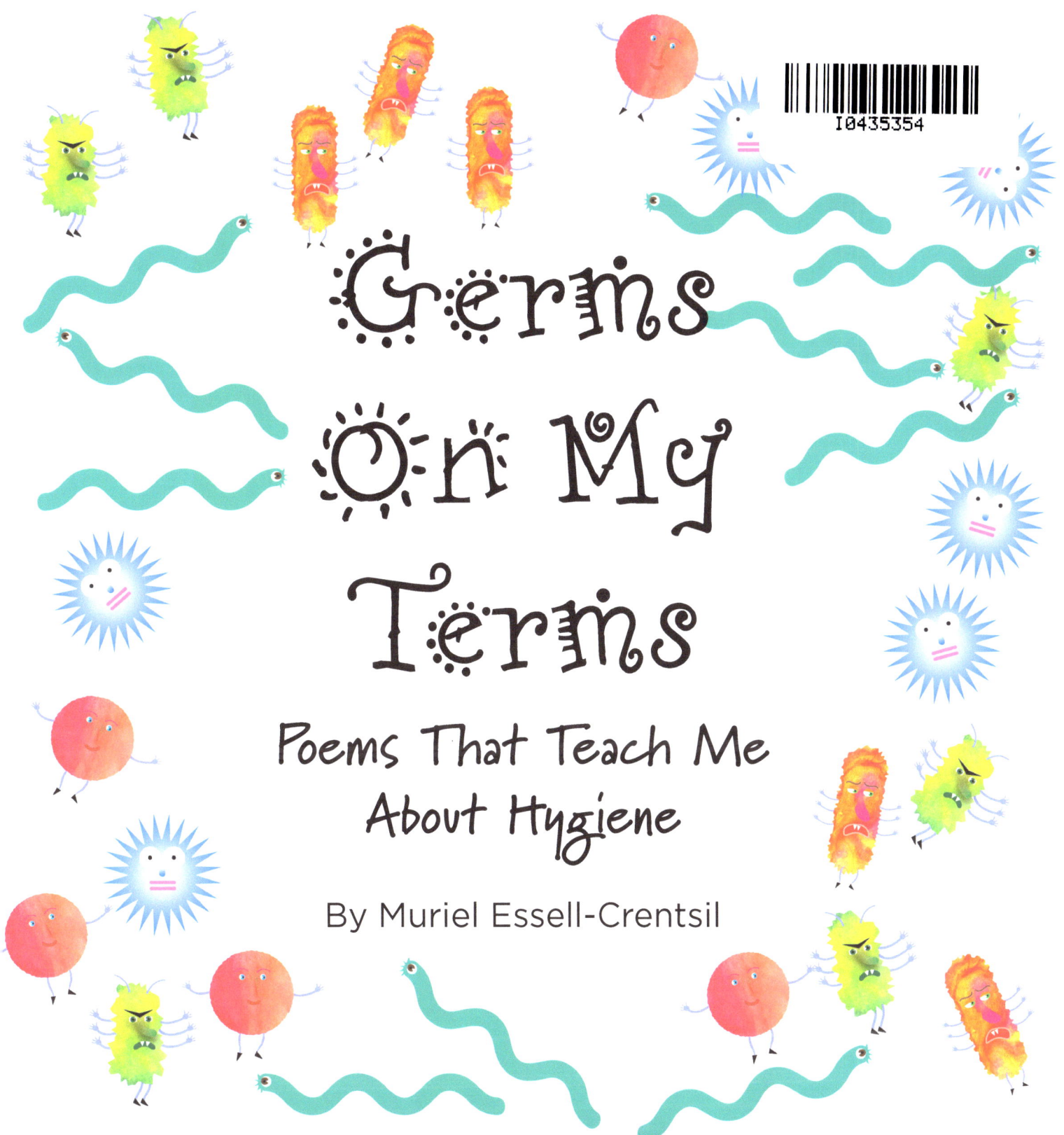

Germs On My Terms

Poems That Teach Me About Hygiene

By Muriel Essell-Crentsil

This Book is Dedicated to My Family Gems

Ab
Paa Kwesi
Lil Joe
Sedzro
Samaria
and
McKayla

This book was inspired by Kwasi Kyei Darkwah (KKD), another logophile, who is also an acclaimed and respected journalist and broadcaster

Acknowledgements

MY GRATITUDE TO THE FOLLOWING:

Martha Galvin, my daughter's very talented 3rd-to-5th grade teacher, who encouraged me to rewrite and rewrite until I got it right.

Markell West, an esteemed editor, for your blessing and golden touch to this book. You are a treasure and a pleasure to work with.

Abigail Tamakloe, my dearest sister and confidante for lending your ears and editor's experience whenever I needed them.

Sheila Crentsil, my beloved stepdaughter— you have an insatiable appetite for reading, and you were there when I needed fresh eyes to look at a sentence or bounce off an idea.

Nana Crentsil, my beloved daughter who has a star in the "reluctant readers' library of fame." The sky is the limit to any endeavor. I understand your teenage rebellion.

Doris Glover Ablo, my friend and adviser who is also a health expert.

Wes Dennis, not only did you tie the nuts and bolts to this book but you also untangled the technological knots with your computer expertise. Even more, I appreciate your literary bits of advice to this piece. I respect your Ivy-League intellect.

Michelle Obama, you are my inspiration. I draw on your passion for a healthier generation to write this maiden book on health.

A big "Thank You" to the students in Summer School 2013 at Ridgecrest Elementary School in Hyattsville, Maryland. It was my pleasure and privilege to read to you.

Kwasi Kyei Darkwah, you are the one who made it all possible. You are the brainchild of this book. Your words to me in 2010: "Muriel, there's a writer in you waiting to be unleashed," still resonate in my dreams.

Good Hygiene for Good Health

For you I write this book on germs,
Which you can fight on your own terms.
This healthy tale for you I tell
With **hygiene** tips to make you well!

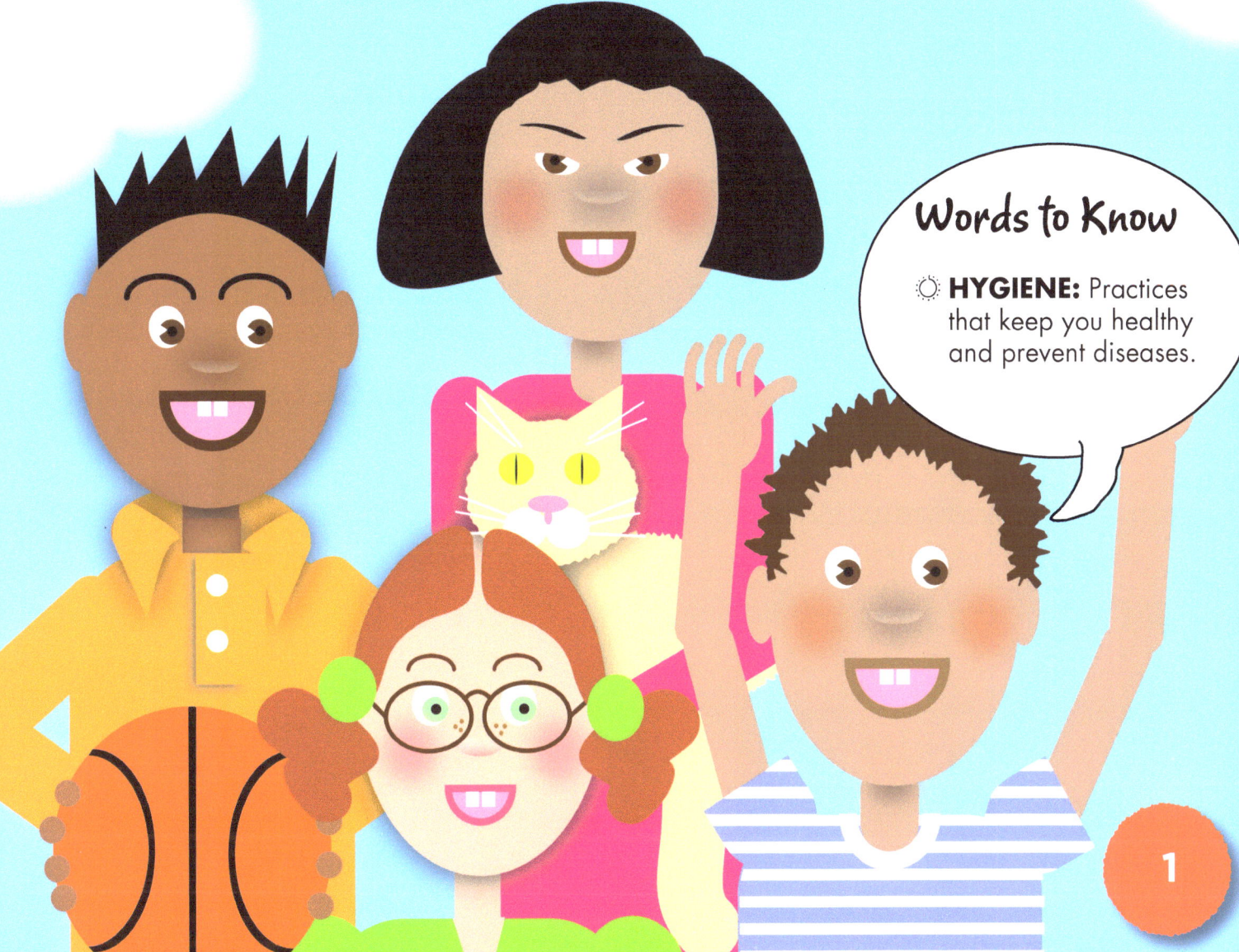

Words to Know

○ **HYGIENE:** Practices that keep you healthy and prevent diseases.

Features of the Creatures Called Germs

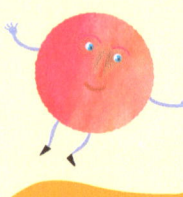

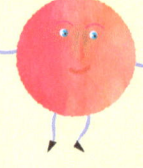

Germs are alive
Germs are tiny
Germs are creatures
See their **features**
In a **microscope**.

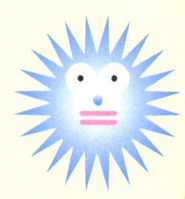

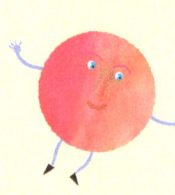

Protozoa and **virus**
Bacteria and **fungus:**
Four big terms
For the types of germs.

Some are harmful
Be aware!
Some are helpful
Let's compare...

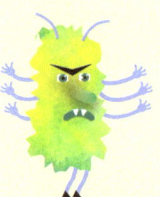

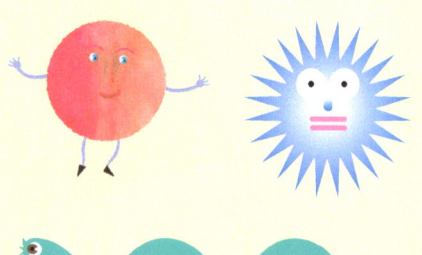

Words to Know

☼ **BACTERIA:** Germs that can cause sore throat, cavities and ear infections.

☼ **FEATURES:** Characteristics, type.

☼ **FUNGUS** (FUNGI–PLURAL): Germs that cause diseases like ringworm and athlete's foot.

☼ **MICROSCOPE:** An instrument used for enlarging very tiny objects.

☼ **PROTOZOA:** Germs that cause diseases like malaria and diarrhea.

☼ **VIRUS** (VIRUSES–PLURAL): A germ that can cause infections like chicken pox and a cold.

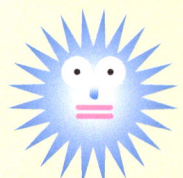

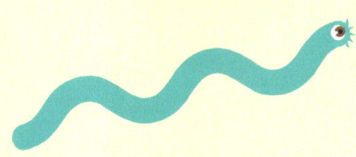

Where the Helpful Germs Are

Healthy germs in yogurt
Healthy germs in the **gut**
Healthy germs help **digestion**
Healthy germs fight **infection**.

Healthy germs make *vaccines*
Healthy germs are unseen
Healthy germs in the *lab*
Healthy germs are so *fab!*

Words to Know

☼ **DIGESTION:** The breakdown of food in the mouth, stomach and intestine.

☼ **GUT:** The stomach, belly or tummy.

☼ **FAB:** Fabulous, wonderful.

☼ **INFECTION:** When germs make us sick.

☼ **LAB (LABORARORY):** A place where scientists perform experiments.

☼ **VACCINE:** Medicines that are made from germs and used as shots to prevent or fight diseases.

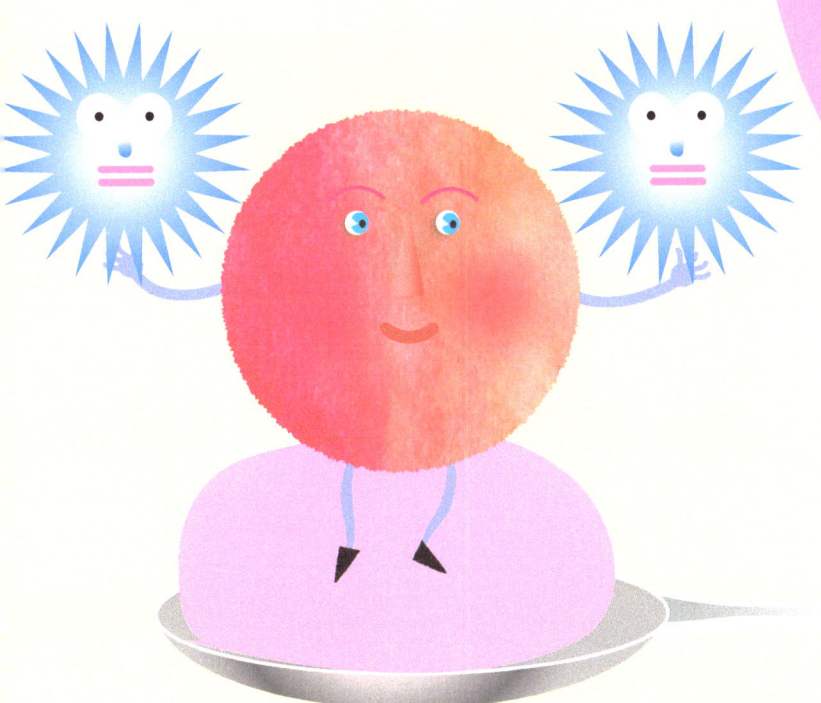

Where the Harmful Germs Are

Germs in our water
Germs really matter
Germs in the mud
Germs in the blood.

Germs in the air
Germs everywhere
Catch germs
   from cats,
Dogs, rats, and bats.

Germs in our zoos
Germs in our shoes
Germs in our nose
Germs on our toes.

Germs in the sink
Germs in a drink
Germs in the sands
Germs on our hands.

We need our vaccines
Before we are teens
So we won't get **mumps**
Or chicken pox bumps.

We need our vaccines
We need our vaccines
Give us our shots
While we are still **tots.**

Words to Know

☼ **MUMPS:** A disease caused by a virus that affects 5- to15-year olds. You will have fever, a swelling and stiffness in front of both ears, the neck and jaws.

☼ **TOT:** A very young child.

4

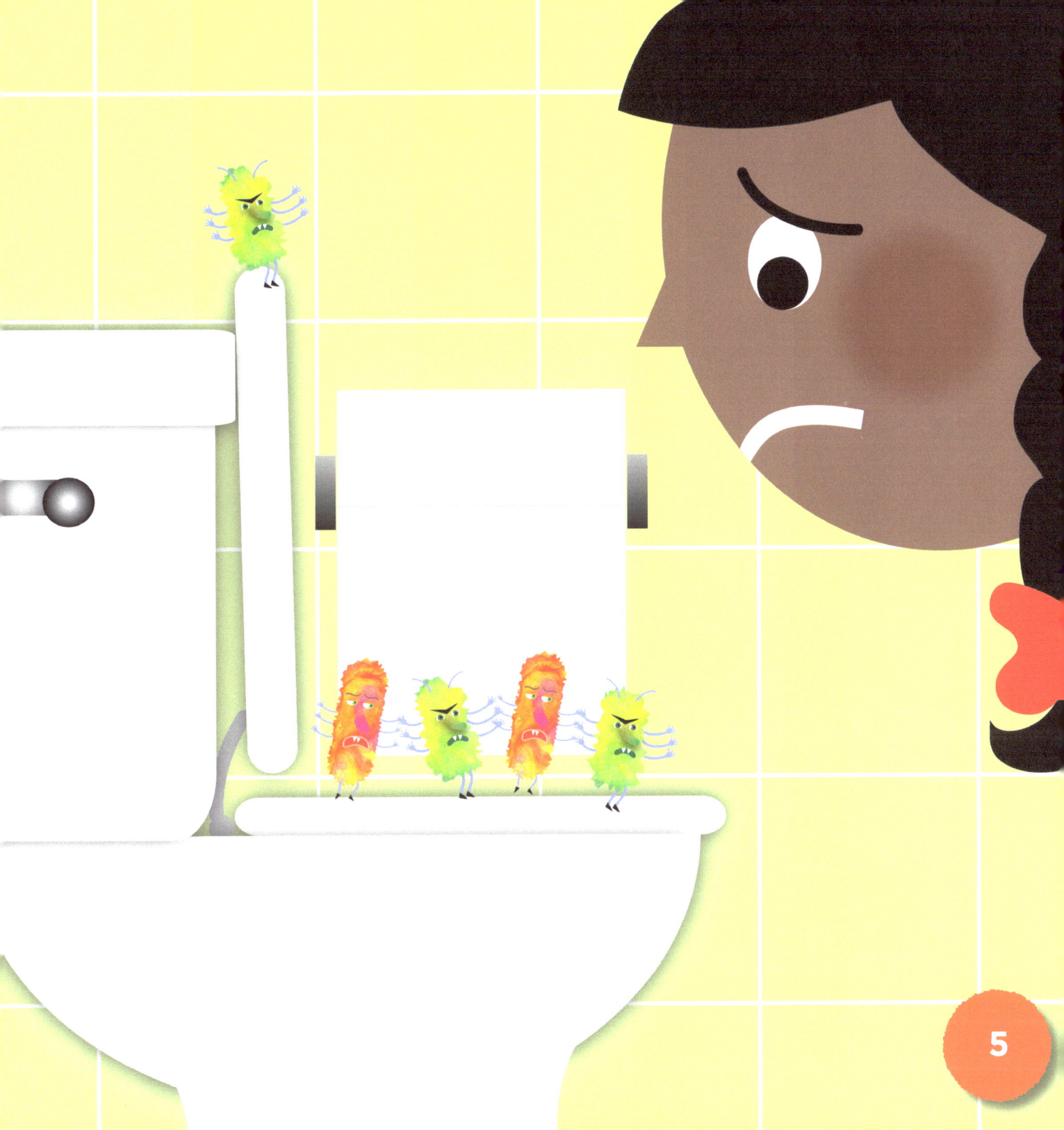

5

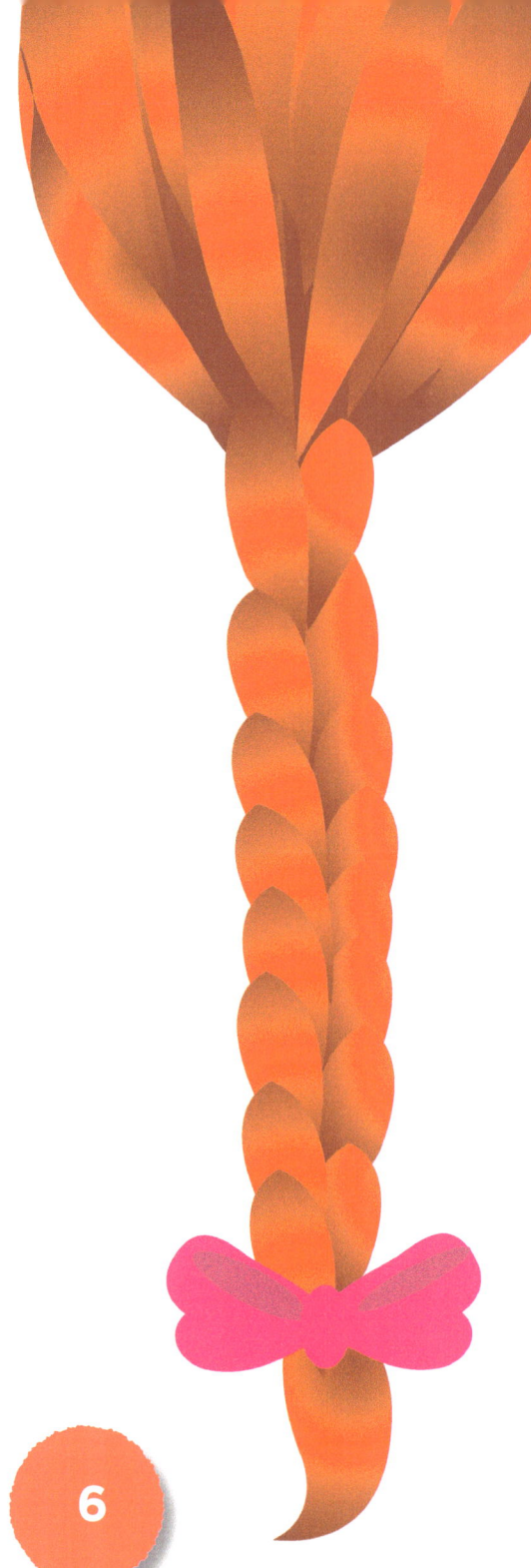

Here's To Healthy Hair

You may wash it every day
You may wash it every week
Either way, wash your hair
Either way, show you care.

Every week
Or every day
Hair that's chic
Can be your way.

Here are tips for healthy hair:
Combs and clips, don't
    you share
For dandruff, ringworm or lice
See a doctor, those aren't nice.

Groom your hair
Show you care
Blond or brown
Love your crown.

Words to Know

CHIC: Stylish, with style.

CROWN: The top of the head.

DANDRUFF: Dry scaly and flaky dead skin from the scalp.

GROOM: To make pretty, to refine.

RINGWORM: A round and itchy rash that is caused by a fungus.

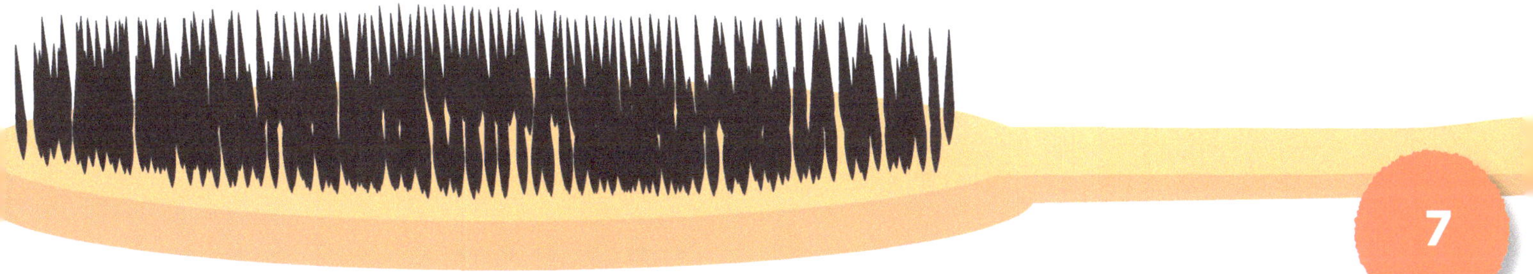

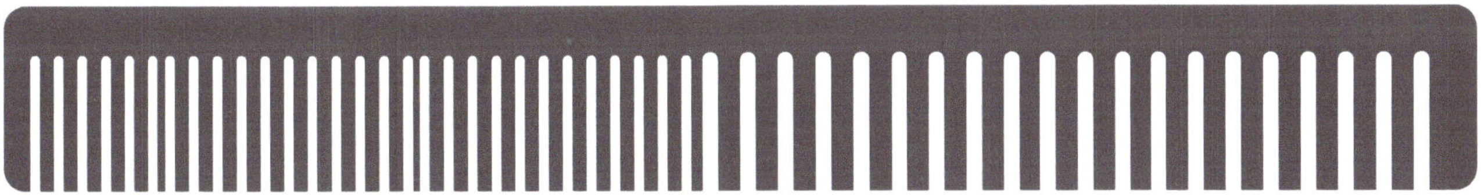

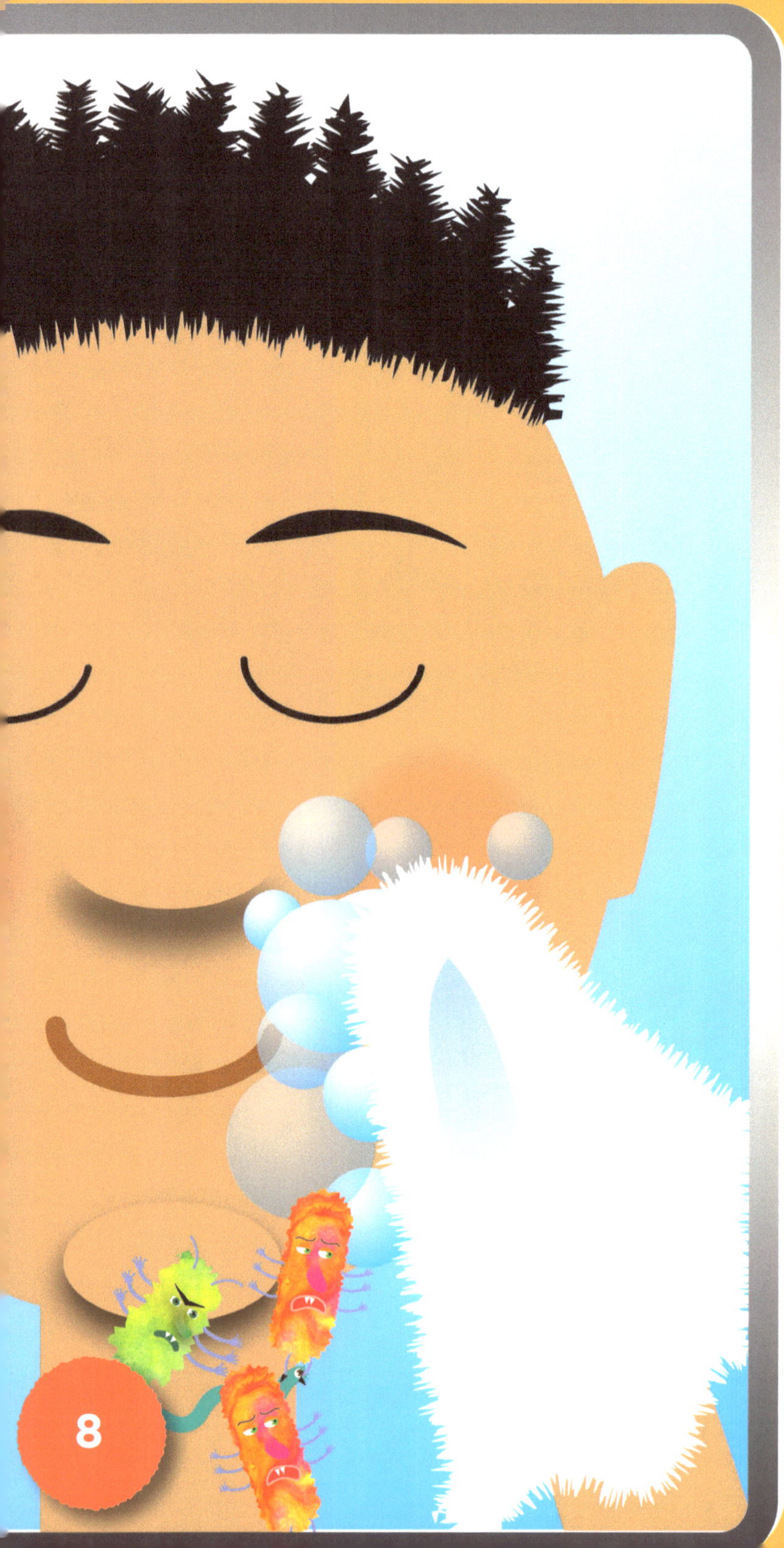

Zap the Harmful Facial Germs

Wash your face
Day and night
Take the time to
Do it right.

After play
Any place
Germs will **sneak**
Onto your face.

Wash your face
Every day
Drive the germs
Far, far away.

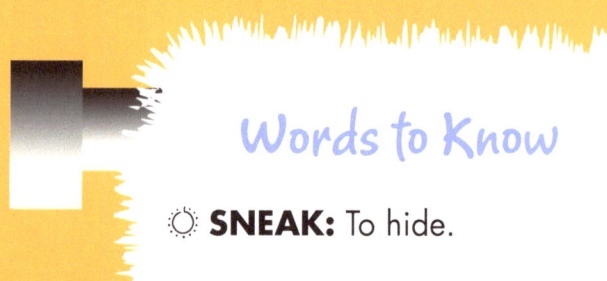

Words to Know

○ **SNEAK:** To hide.

○ **ZAP:** To destroy or kill.

8

Protect Your Eyes

Keep the **sparkle**
If you're wise
Keep your hands
Off of your eyes.

Hear my reason
And my **rhyme:**
Wash your hands
All the time.

Clean your lenses
Will you please?
Clean those glasses
Stop disease.

If you have pain in your eye
See a doctor, don't **delay**
If there's swelling and a **sty**
See a doctor right away.

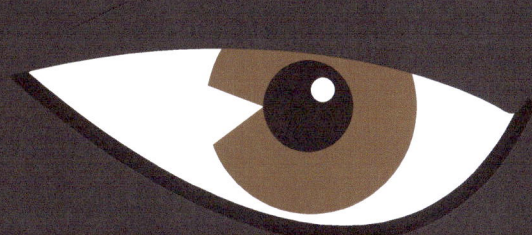
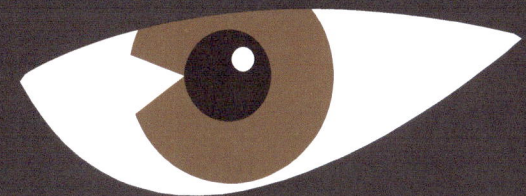

WORDS TO KNOW

○ **DELAY:** To wait.

○ **RHYME:** A word that agrees in sound with another.

○ **SPARKLE:** Something that shines.

○ **STY (STYES—PLURAL):** A red, and painful bump on the eyelid caused by bacteria.

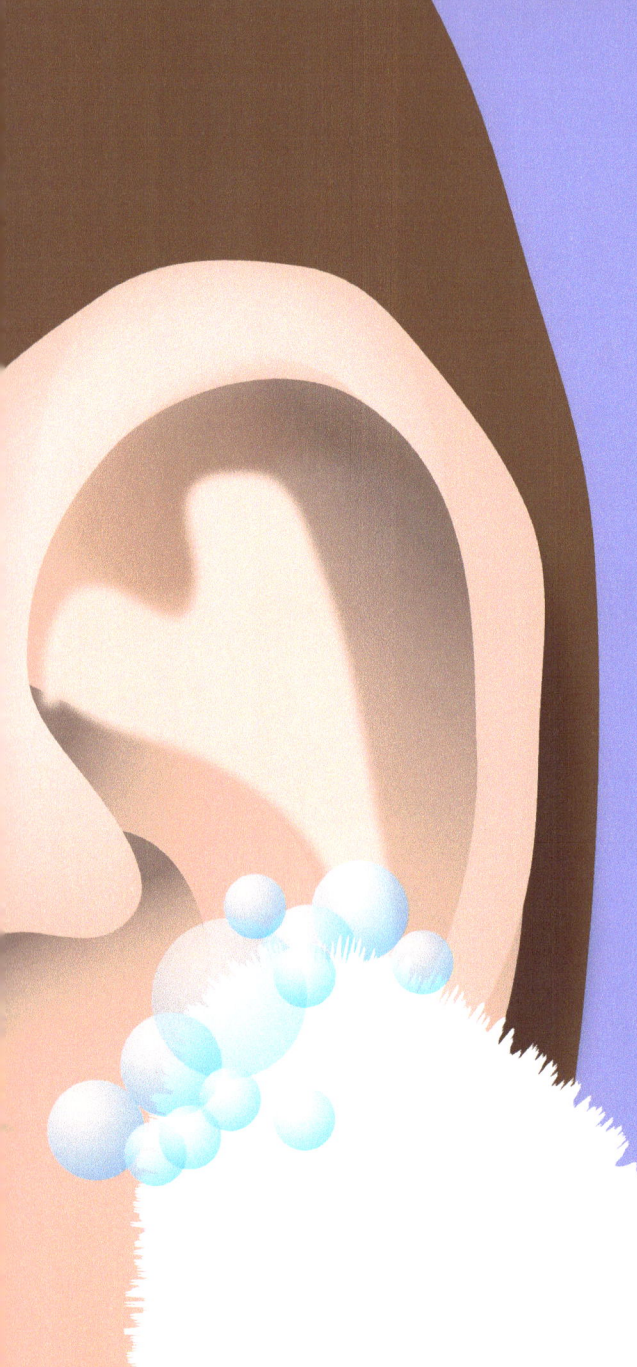

Protect Your Hearing: Clean Your Ears!

Here's the way to clean your ear:
Soap and water you will need
Wipe the outer ear 'til clean
This advice I hope you **heed**.

Being **deaf,** you must fear
Things like Q-Tips you must **toss**
Don't need a thing inside your ear
If you don't want hearing loss.

Your earphones, I hope you know
Are meant for you alone
They carry many unseen germs
Your **peers** should have their own.

Earphones carry germs **galore**
Clean your earphones every day
Though the germs you
cannot see
Clean your earphones
anyway.

If you choose to *pierce* your ears
This is what you need to know
Messy pus on your earlobe?
Clean it well, don't say "no."

Drainage, *blockage* in your ear?
That's a matter of *concern*
If there's pain and you can't hear
Then your doctor should *discern*.

If you don't hear robins sing
Ask your doctor, not your boss
If you hear your *eardrums* ring
Maybe you have hearing loss.

WORDS TO KNOW

☼ **BLOCKAGE:** Wax build-up that can block the ear canal and may cause hearing loss.

☼ **CONCERN:** Worry or bother.

☼ **DISCERN:** To see, understand or recognize.

☼ **DEAF:** Unable to hear.

☼ **DRAINAGE:** Fluid from the ear.

☼ **EARDRUM:** A part of the middle ear that is important for hearing.

☼ **GALORE:** A lot, many.

☼ **HEED:** To listen, pay attention.

☼ **PEER:** Pal, friend.

☼ **PIERCE:** To make a hole.

☼ **TOSS:** To throw away.

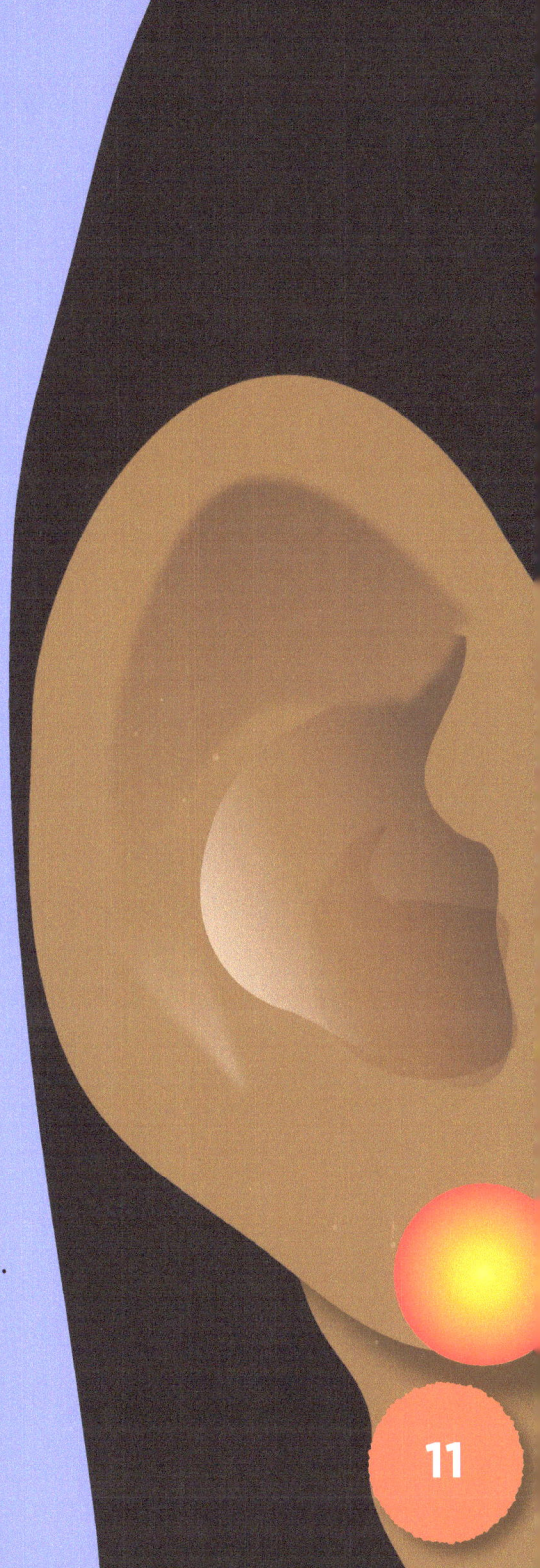

Don't Spread Germs
From Your Mouth, Nose & Throat

Virus, fungus, bacteria...
Bacteria causes **listeria**
Those germs called protozoa
Are **parasites** of **malaria.**

Germs may come into your throat
In the air they always float
Germs may come inside your nose
They may hide out on your toes.

In our water and our food
Germs will sneak; some aren't good
They may hide out on the floor
Or the knob of a door.

They swim in your pool
And rule in our school
They are on our hands
In the soil and the sands.

You can catch them from the air
You can catch them from a chair
Slick germs here and there
Sick germs everywhere.

When your throat is red and sore
Do not spit **phlegm** on the floor
Use some tissue, show you care
Use the trash can over there!

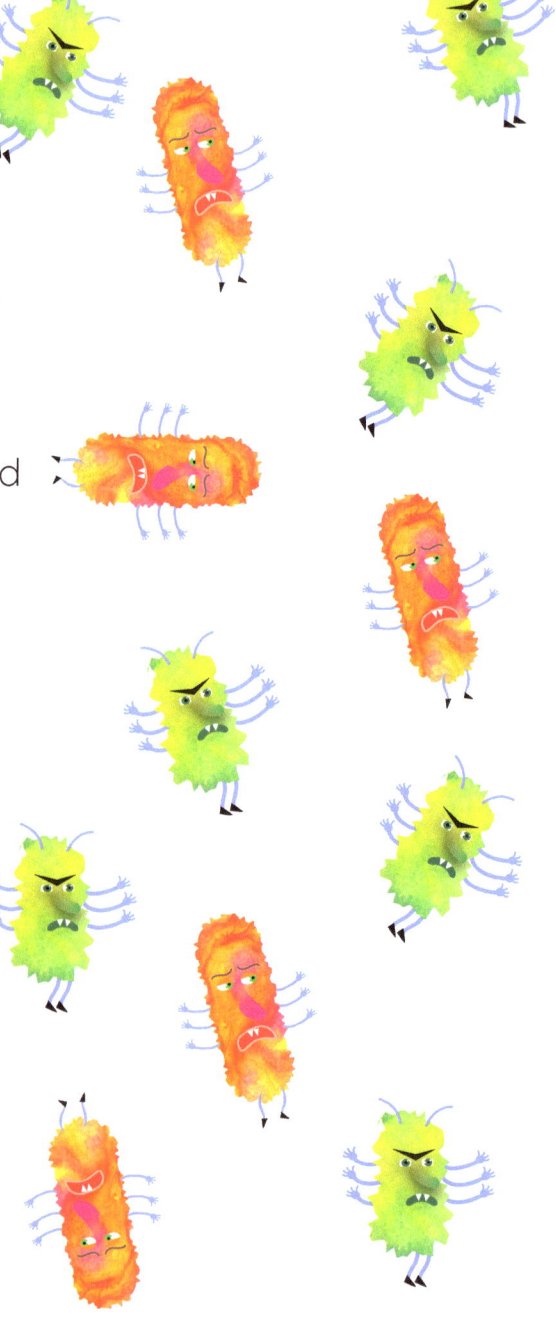

When you cough and cough and cough
You should take a few days off
If you care, take a stand
Do not cough into your hand.

Just in case you need to sneeze
Use some tissue or your sleeve
Do not sneeze into the air
Spreading germs isn't fair.

If your nose you have to blow
This is what you need to know:
Spreading germs is an issue
Blow your nose into a tissue.

Countless times you must wash:
The only way you can *quash*
The many germs on your hands
Against germs, take a stand.

WORDS TO KNOW

☼ **LISTERIA:** A disease that you get from contaminated food.

☼ **MALARIA:** A disease found in hot areas that is spread by mosquito bites.

☼ **PARASITE:** A plant or animal that feeds on another plant or animal

☼ **PHLEGM:** Thick, sticky mucus from the lungs that comes out of your nose or mouth when you have a cold.

☼ **QUASH:** To cancel, suppress, or put an end to.

☼ **SLICK:** Sneaky or slippery.

13

Hygiene for Good Dental Health

Brush your teeth
Twice at least:
When you wake,
Or after a feast
"Do it right,"
Say your mums,
"Brush your teeth,
Your tongue and gums."

Brush and floss,
Between your gums
Stop tooth loss
And zap tooth scum
Brush your teeth
Front and back
Round and round
After a snack.

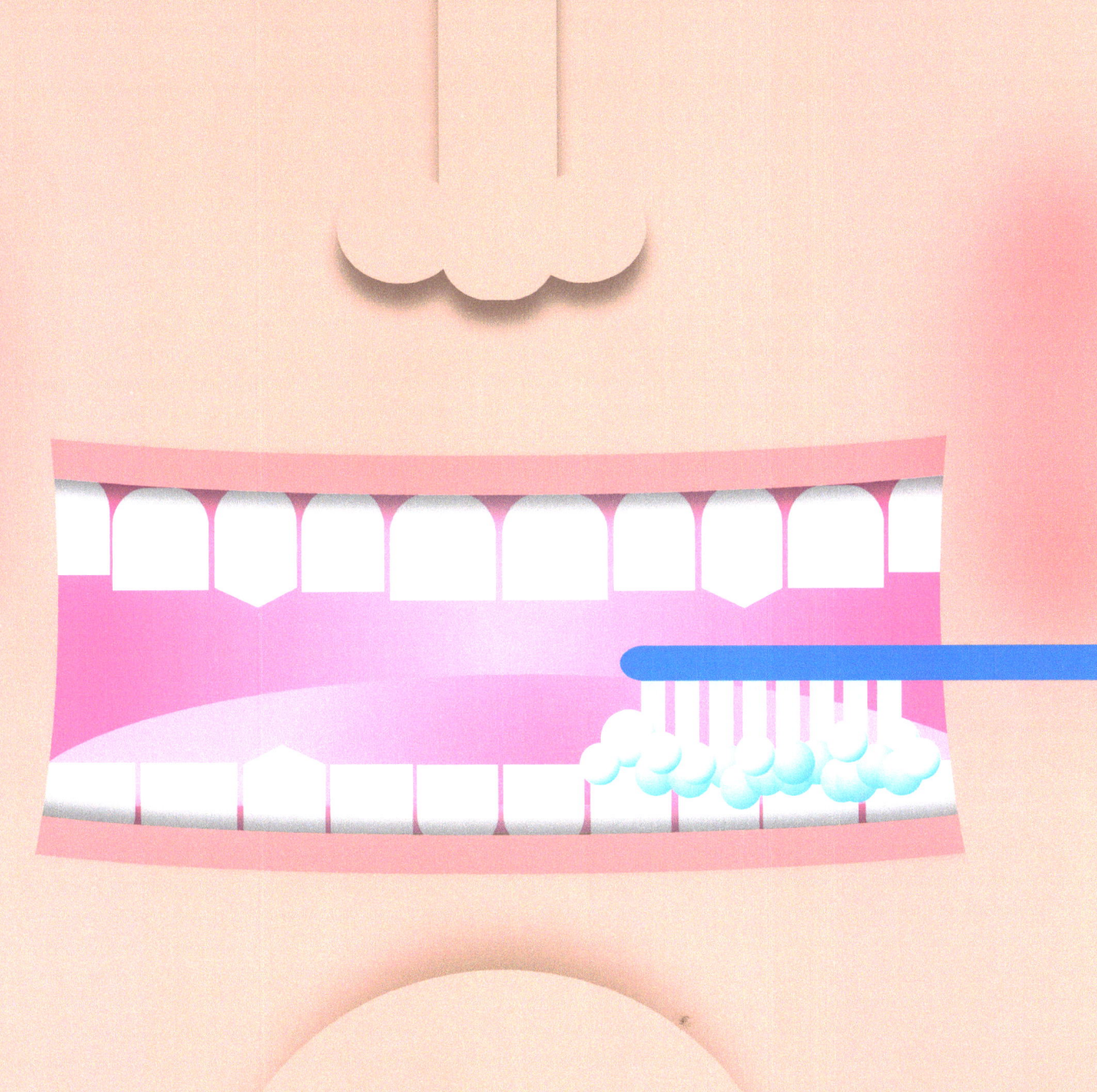

Baby Dental Care

After a nap and after they eat
Newborns need some mouth care too
Wet a soft cloth and clean their mouths
Don't you wait 'til they turn two!

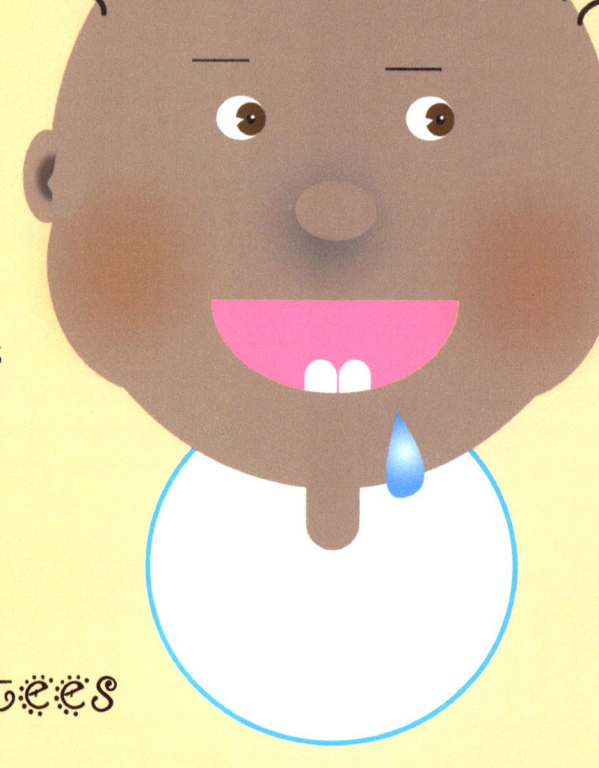

Good Nutrition Guarantees Good Dentition

Calcium helps your bones and teeth:
Calcium-rich foods you must eat
Help prevent that tooth disease
Reach for milk or yogurt treats.

Some cheese is good
If you don't overeat
Vegetables are good
If you don't overheat.

Toothpaste Choice & Toothbrush Care

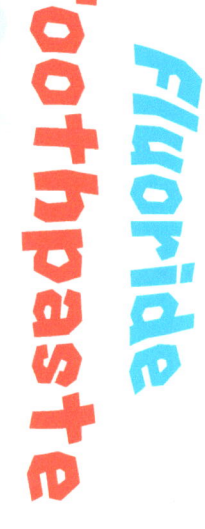

A soft-bristle brush: the best to choose
Fluoride toothpaste: the best to use
Rinse your mouth and change your brush
Or in three months you might get **thrush.**

Brush and **floss** and use mouthwash:
Bacteria and fungus you can quash
If your teeth you do not brush,
Fungus and germs you cannot crush.

Watch Those Treats

Tobacco, and coffee
Your teeth may **stain**
May cause bad breath
Or **strain** your brain.

Mind the sweets and the sodas
They breed germs, watch your **quota**.

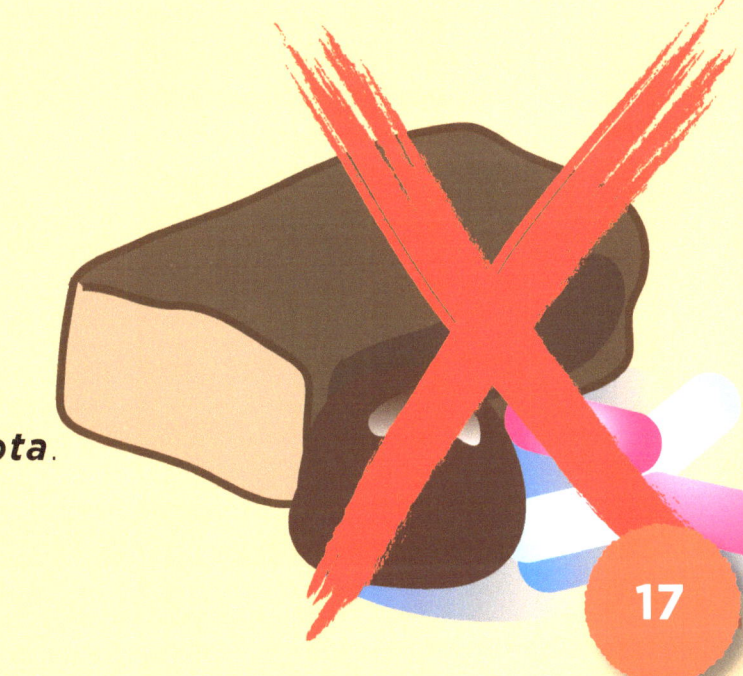

17

DENTIST'S OFFICE

WORDS TO KNOW

☼ **CALCIUM:** A mineral that supports healthy teeth and bones.

☼ **CAVITIES:** Hole in the teeth that can cause toothaches and bad breath.

☼ **DECAY:** Spoil, rotten.

☼ **DENTITION:** The makeup of a set of teeth.

 ☼ **FLOSS:** A dental thread for cleaning between the teeth.

☼ **FLUORIDE:** A mineral that promotes healthy teeth and prevents tooth decay.

☼ **QUOTA:** A share amount.

☼ **SCUM:** Dirt.

☼ **STAIN:** Discolor.

☼ **STRAIN:** Damage, stress.

☼ **THRUSH**: A fungus infection of the mouth and tongue.

Visiting the Dentist

Gingivitis is gum disease
Cavities are tooth **decay**
Halitosis is bad breath.
See a dentist, don't delay.

Visit the dentist
Twice a year
She'll clean your teeth
Your smile will cheer.

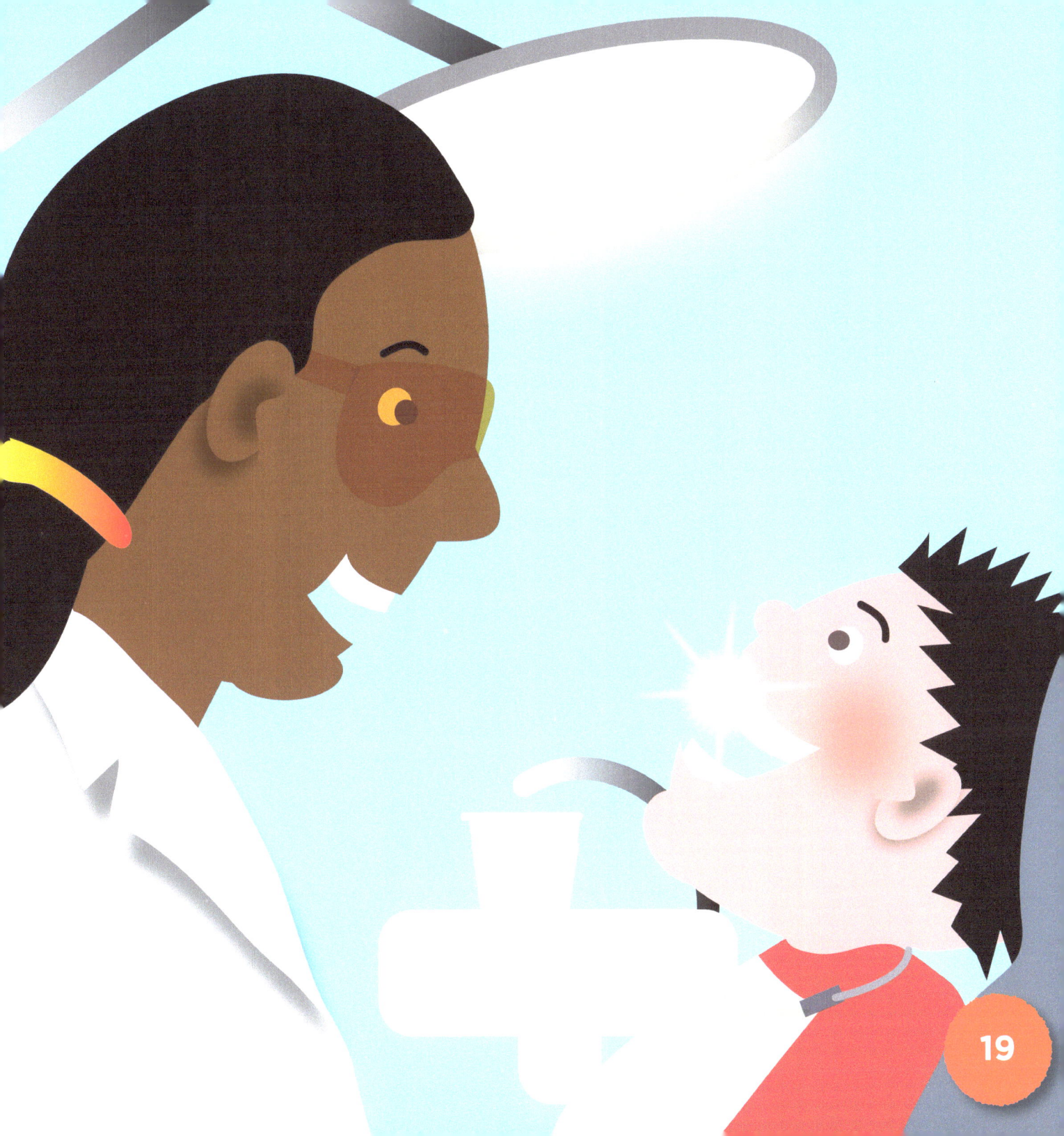

19

Hand Washing Wins the War on Germs

A million germs
Live on our hands
And here's the reason why:

Before we eat
After we eat
We have to wash our hands.

Before we cook
Can't overlook
We have to wash our hands.

When we blow our nose
Or touch our toes
We have to wash our hands.

When we touch our pet
We can't forget
We have to wash our hands.

When we visit the sick
Germs we can kick
If we will wash our hands.

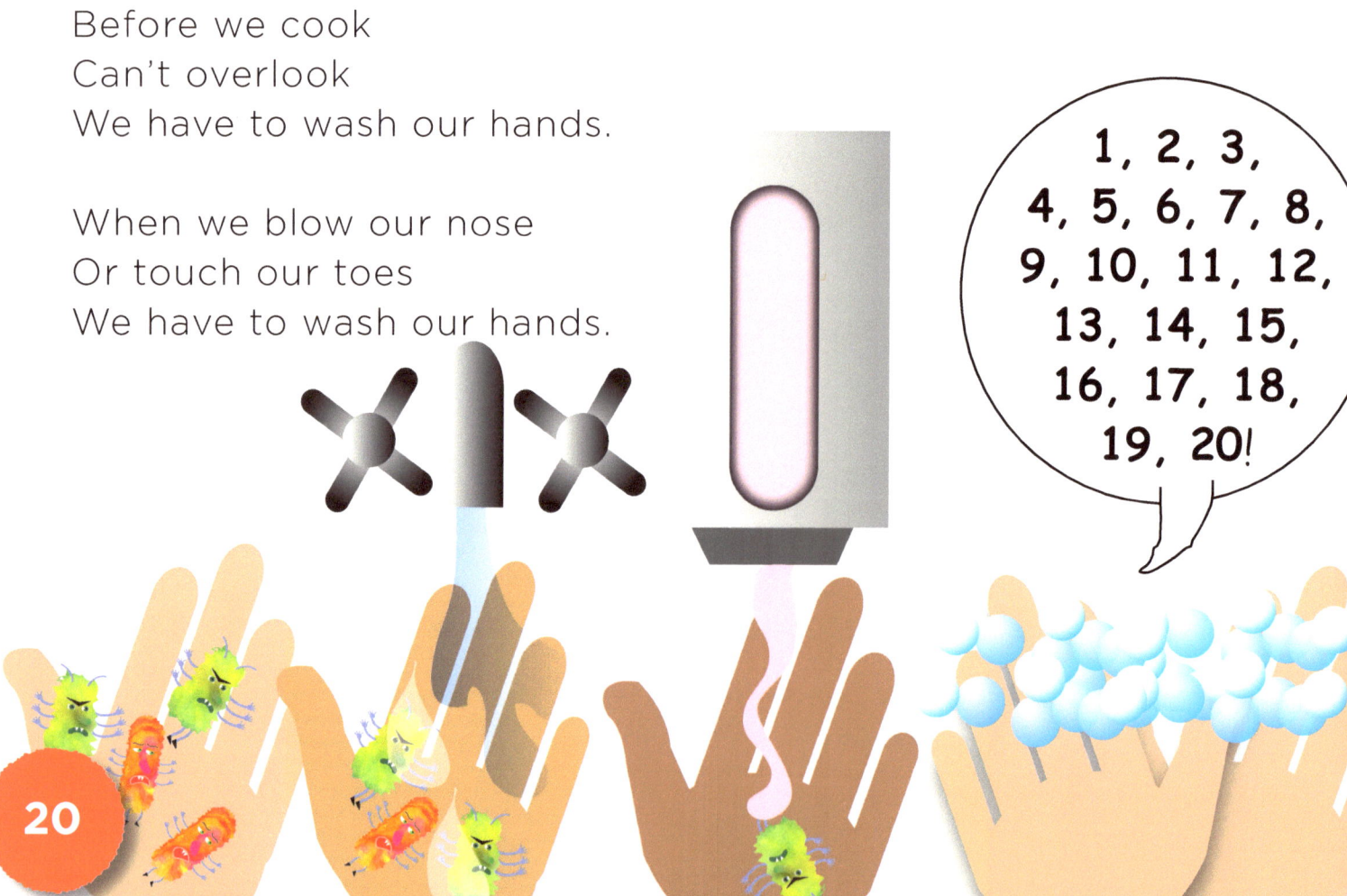

1, 2, 3,
4, 5, 6, 7, 8,
9, 10, 11, 12,
13, 14, 15,
16, 17, 18,
19, 20!

20

After we **urinate**
Shouldn't **hesitate**
We have to wash our hands.

With water and soap, our hands we scrub
For 20 seconds, our hands we rub:
The way to wash our hands.

Now we're **convinced**
Our hands must be rinsed
After we've washed our hands:

Our hands we'll dry
And say goodbye
To the germs on our hands.

WORDS TO KNOW

○ **CONVINCE:** To make someone believe, to prove, or to persuade.

○ **HESITATE:** Wait to act, have doubt.

○ **URINATE:** Pass urine, to pee.

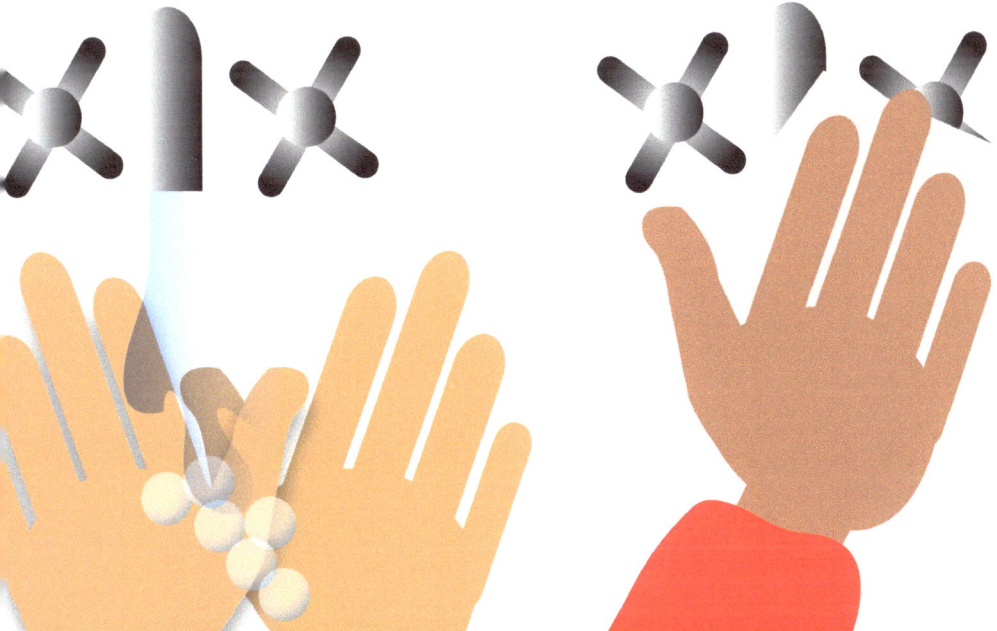

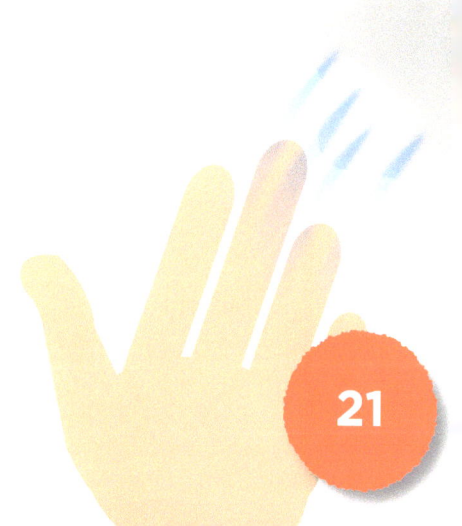

21

Don't Bite Your Nails

Don't bite your nails
Females and males
Germs will crawl in
If you break your skin
With dirty tricks
They'll make you sick.

Long nails are nice
Germs they **entice**
Germs can be mean
Keep your nails clean
Keep your nails **trim**
And proper and **prim**.

22

Look and Smell Good

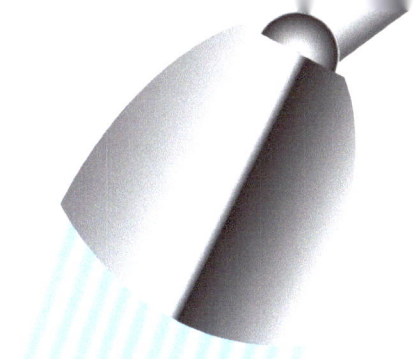

Sweat and bacteria cause body **odor**
That makes you smell so bad
Your friends at school may laugh at you
And make you feel so sad.

Bye-bye ***bromhidrosis***
See you later, halitosis!
Brush your teeth! stop halitosis
Take a bath! Stop bromhidrosis.

Disease or ***drugs*** and certain foods
Will make you smell bad too
Pay attention to your hygiene
That's what you need to do.

Watch the ***seasonings***
Mind the ***spices***
Smell like spice
What a price!

To body odor, just say, "No!"
Take a shower every day
This is what you need to know:
Sweat and germs will wash away.

Dry yourself after you shower
Deodorize each underarm
Wear clean clothes and underwear
Look and smell good: show your charm!

WORDS TO KNOW

○ **BROMHIDROSIS:** Body odor.

○ **DEODORIZE:** Get rid of unpleasant odor.

○ **DRUGS:** Medicine.

○ **ODOR:** A bad or pleasant smell or scent

○ **SEASONING:** Food additives that add flavor and aroma to food.

○ **SPICE:** Substances used for flavoring food, such as pepper and mint.

23

Beat Feet Germs

Take care of your feet and toes
You must wash them every day
If you think they do not sweat
You must wash them anyway.

Air out sweaty feet and toes
Wash and dry them very well
Don't wear plastic or tight shoes
They can cause your feet to smell.

Germs love dirty socks and shoes
Wear some clean socks every day
Make sure that your shoes are clean
Before you put them all away.

Germs live underneath your shoes
So leave them at the door
Scores of germs are on the floor
Mopping must be a chore.

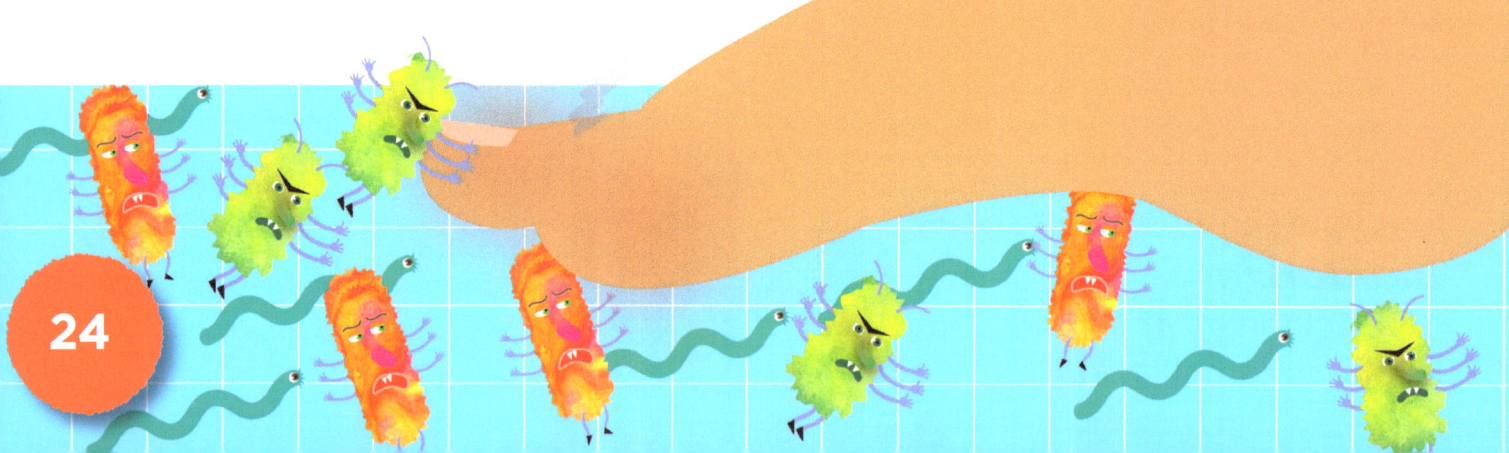

Don't go barefoot 'round the pool
Athletes, "watch the locker room."
These are homes for
athlete's foot
Where fungi like to lounge
and **loom**.

In case you get athlete's foot
Find a **pharmacist** who knows
An anti-fungal cream to buy
That will heal your feet and toes.

Podiatrists care for our toes
and feet
So find one you can see
For many problems on your feet
You'll be **infection**-free.

WORDS TO KNOW

☼ **ATHLETE'S FOOT:** Ringworm of the foot also known as *tinea pedis.*

☼ **INFECTION:** When bad germs cause sickness.

☼ **LOOM:** To appear in a scary way.

☼ **PHARMACIST:** A person trained and licensed to prepare and sell medicines.

☼ **PODIATRIST:** A doctor trained to treat foot diseases.

First Lady's Lasting Legacy

First Lady, we know you care
We do embrace the words you share
Obesity is what we'll fight
With exercise and eating right.

Obesity—our children's plight
You took a stand; and said, "Let's fight."
Obesity—we'll stamp it out
With healthy ways, there is no doubt.

Play some music; it's time to dance!
Let's have some fun, our health **enhance**
We'll jump up high, a ball to **clutch**
And on the ground we'll **double dutch.**

First Lady, you are **graceful**
Mrs. Obama, we are **grateful**
You **inspire** us with all you do
First Lady, we **salute** you!

WORDS TO KNOW

○ **CLUTCH:** To grasp and hold tightly.

○ **DOUBLE DUTCH:** A rope-skipping exercise using two ropes.

○ **ENHANCE:** Build up.

○ **GRACEFUL:** Beauty or elegance of manner.

○ **GRATEFUL:** Thankful.

○ **INSPIRE:** To influence in a positive way.

○ **OBESITY:** A medical conditi in which one gains excessive body fat that affects health.

○ **PLIGHT:** Trouble or difficulty

○ **SALUTE:** To show respect.

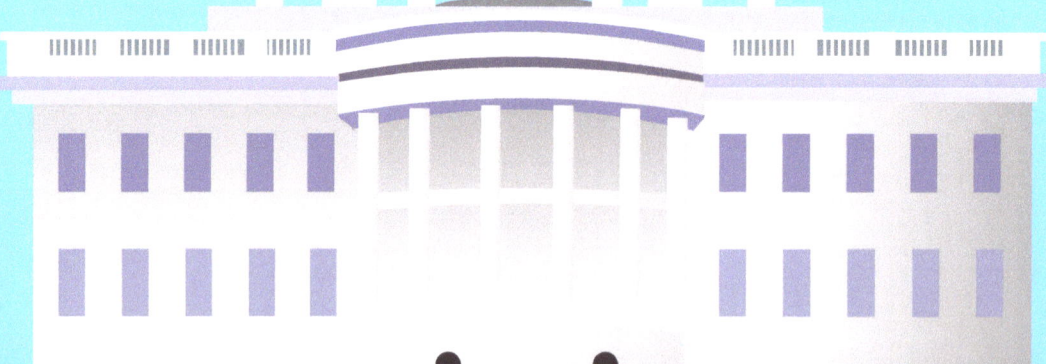

Healthy Habits That Fight Disease

Good hygiene disease will fight
It also helps to eat just right
Sanitize and *immunize*
Rest and sleep and exercise.

Hope you take this health advice
Makes you healthy and more wise!

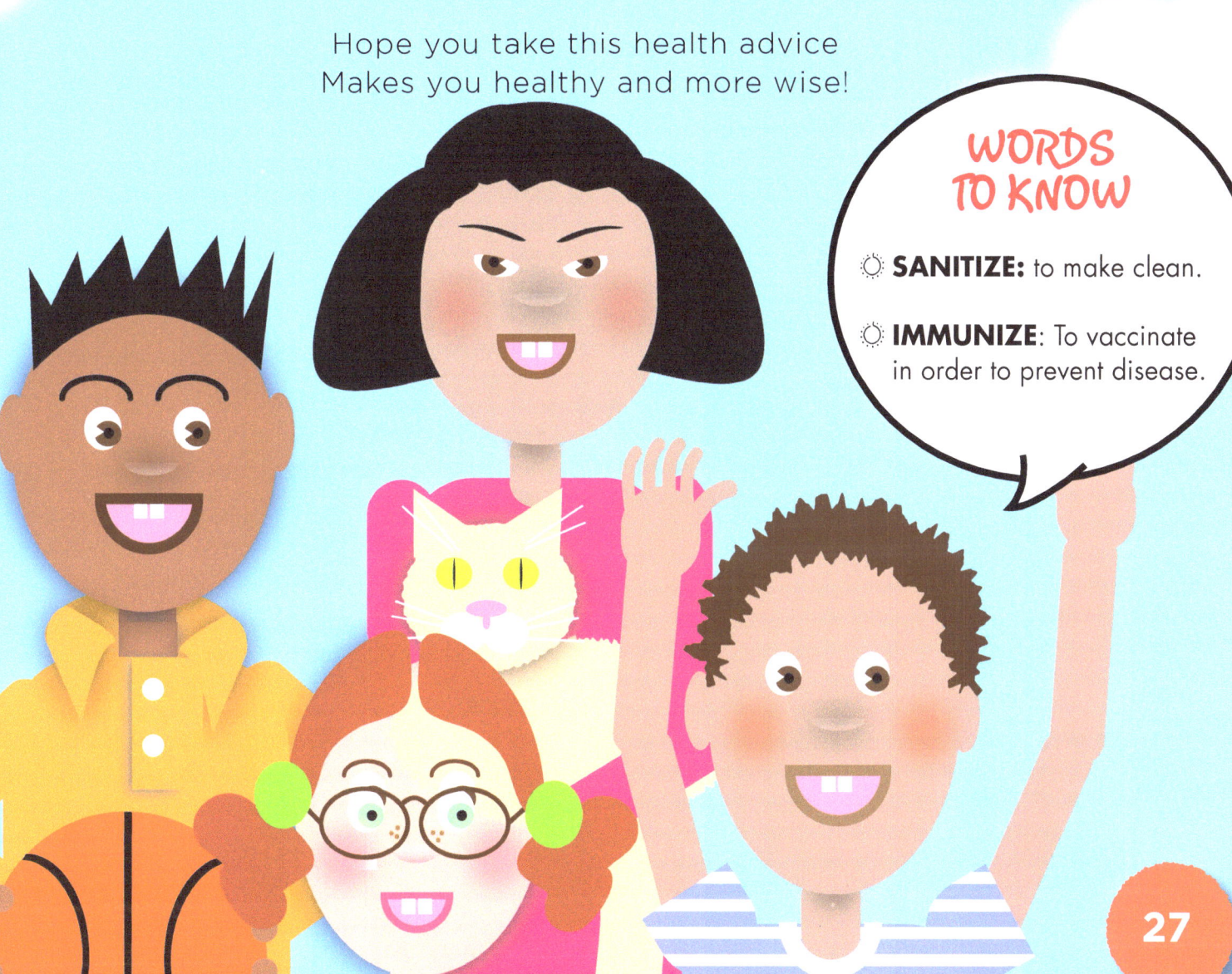

WORDS TO KNOW

○ **SANITIZE:** to make clean.

○ **IMMUNIZE**: To vaccinate in order to prevent disease.

27

Extra Words

AUDIOLOGIST: A person trained to diagnose & treat hearing and balance problems.

BRUXISM: Grinding of teeth.

CONJUNCTIVITIS: Also called "pinkeye," is an inflammation or infection of the white part of the eye, that causes redness, tears, blurred vision, burning, itching and green or white discharge.

CRADLE CAP: Infant seborrhea or dandruff.

DEODORANT: A substance that you rub or spray in your armpit to control sweat and bad odor.

DERMATOLOGIST: A doctor who takes care of skin diseases.

EPISTAXIS: Nose-bleed

LINGUA: A tongue

MANICURE: Take care of the hands and fingernails

MYOPIA: Nearsightedness or the ability to see objects that are near better than those that are far away.

OPHTHALMOLOGIST: A medical doctor who specializes in eye and vision care and can perform surgery.

OPTICIAN: Uses the prescription from an eye doctor to fit and sell eye glasses and contact lenses. Some opticians have formal training but some do not.

OPTOMETRIST: An eye doctor who has a degree in optometry and can give eye and vision care, but cannot perform eye surgery.

ORAL: By word of mouth. Spoken or related to speech.

ORTHODONTIST: A dentist who treats people with crooked teeth and face. He uses braces to help straighten the teeth.

PEDICULOSIS: A condition of having lice, which are insects that live on the human body or hair and feed on blood.

PEDICURE: Professional care of the feet and toenails

PERIODONTAL DISEASE: Bacterial infections that affect the gums and bones of the teeth.

PRESBYCUSIS: Hearing loss that occurs gradually as people age.

PRESBYOPIA: Farsightedness or the ability to see objects that are far better and cannot see objects that are close well.

RHINITIS: Runny nose with an irritation and inflammation of the lining of the nose.

SEBORRHEA: Red itchy rash and white scales that is called dandruff when it is on the scalp. It can also be on the face, chest, under arms, below the breasts, groin and buttocks.

TINNITUS: Ringing in the ear.

www.ingramcontent.com/pod-product-compliance
Lightning Source LLC
Chambersburg PA
CBHW041535280526
45792CB00004B/1512